CW00505700

The Complete Instant Pot Cookbook For Beginners

Pressure Cooker Recipes For Affordable Homemade Meals

Jacklyn Moore

© Copyright 2021 - All rights reserved.

The content contained within this book may not be reproduced, duplicated or transmitted without direct written permission from the author or the publisher.

Under no circumstances will any blame or legal responsibility be held against the publisher, or author, for any damages, reparation, or monetary loss due to the information contained within this book. Either directly or indirectly.

Legal Notice:

This book is copyright protected. This book is only for personal use. You cannot amend, distribute, sell, use, quote or paraphrase any part, or the content within this book, without the consent of the author or publisher.

Disclaimer Notice:

Please note the information contained within this document is for educational and entertainment purposes only. All effort has been executed to present accurate, up to date, and reliable, complete information. No warranties of any kind are declared or implied. Readers acknowledge that the author is not engaging in the rendering of legal, financial, medical or professional advice. The content within this book has been derived from various sources. Please consult a licensed professional before attempting any techniques outlined in this book.

By reading this document, the reader agrees that under no circumstances is the author responsible for any losses, direct or indirect, which are incurred as a result of the use of information contained within this document, including, but not limited to, — errors, omissions, or inaccuracies.

Sommario

Introduction

This complete as well as helpful overview to immediate pot cooking with over 1000 recipes for breakfast, supper, dinner, and even desserts! This is just one of the most extensive split second pot recipe books ever before released thanks to its range as well as accurate   guidelines. Innovative dishes and also standards, modern take on family members's most loved meals-- all this is yummy, basic and also naturally as healthy as it can be. Adjustment the way you prepare with these ingenious split second pot guidelines. Need a brand-new supper or a treat? Here you are! Finest instant pot dishes collaborated in a few simple steps, even a novice can do it! The instantaneous pot defines the means you cook on a daily basis. This instantaneous pot cookbook assists you make the absolute most   out   of   your   regular   menu. The only split second pot book you will ever before need with the best collection of dishes will help you towards a simpler as well as much healthier cooking area experience. If you want to conserve time cooking meals more efficiently, if you intend to provide your household food that can please also the pickiest eater, you remain in the right area! Master your split second pot and also make your food preparation requires suit your busy way of living.

Side Dishes

Cayenne Green Beans

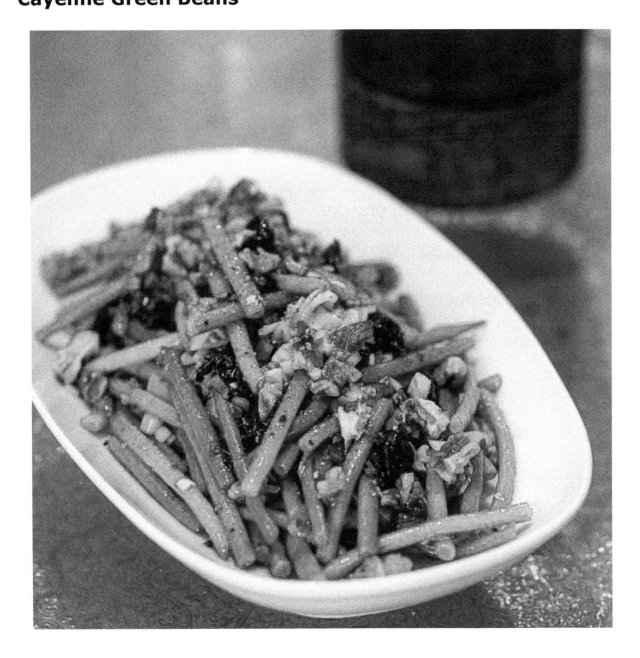

Prep time: 10 minutes

Cooking time: 15 minutes

Servings: 8

Ingredients:

- 12 ounces green beans

- 1 teaspoon garlic powder

- 1 teaspoon onion powder

- 4 garlic cloves

- 2 tablespoons olive oil

- 1 teaspoon cayenne pepper

- 1 jalapeno pepper

- 1 teaspoon butter

- ½ teaspoon salt

- 1 cup of water

Directions:

1. Wash the green beans and cut each into two equal parts.

2. Toss the green beans in the mixing bowl. Sprinkle the vegetables with the onion powder, chili pepper, and salt and stir.

3. Remove the seeds from the jalapeno pepper and chop it into tiny pieces. Add the chopped jalapeno in the green beans mixture.

4. Peel the garlic and slice it. Combine the sliced garlic with the olive oil. Blend the mixture and transfer it to the pressure cooker. Add the water and stir.

5. Put the green beans in the pressure cooker and close the lid. Set the pressure cooker mode to "Sauté," and cook the vegetables for 15 minutes.

6. When the dish is cooked, you should have firm but not crunchy green beans.

7. Remove the green beans from the pressure cooker and discard the liquid before serving.

Nutrition: calories 49, fat 4.1, fiber 1, carbs 3, protein 1

Parmesan Tomatoes

Prep time: 7 minutes

Cooking time: 7 minutes

Servings: 5

Ingredients:

- 10 ounces big tomatoes
- 7 ounces Parmesan cheese
- ½ teaspoon paprika
- 3 tablespoons olive oil
- 1 tablespoon basil
- 1 teaspoon cilantro
- 1 teaspoon onion powder

Directions:

1. Wash the tomatoes and slice them into the thick slices.

2. Spray the pressure cooker with the olive oil inside. Transfer the tomato slices in the pressure cooker.

3. Combine the paprika, basil, and cilantro together and mix well. Grate the Parmesan cheese and sprinkle the tomato slices with the cheese and spice mixture.

4. Close the pressure cooker lid and cook on the "Sauté" mode for 7 minutes.

5. When the cooking time ends, open the pressure cooker lid and let the tomatoes rest briefly. Transfer the dish to the serving plate.

Nutrition: calories 250, fat 19.3, fiber 1, carbs 7.85, protein 12

Mustard Bok Choy

Prep time: 10 minutes

Cooking time: 12 minutes

Servings: 7

Ingredients:

- 1 pound bok choy
- 1 cup of water
- ⅓ cup of soy sauce
- 1 teaspoon salt
- 1 teaspoon red chili flakes
- 5 tablespoon mustard
- ⅓ cup cream
- 1 teaspoon cumin seeds
- 1 teaspoon ground black pepper
- 1 tablespoon butter
- ¼ cup garlic clove

Directions:

1. Wash the bok choy and chop it into pieces.

2. Combine water, soy sauce, salt, chili flakes, cumin seeds, and ground black pepper together. Blend the mixture.

3. Peel the garlic clove and cut into thin slices.

4. Add the butter in the pressure cooker and sliced garlic.

5. Set the pressure cooker to "Sauté" mode and sauté for 1 minute. Add the cream, soy sauce mixture, and bok choy. Close the lid.

6. Set the pot to «Sauté» mode and cook for 10 minutes.

7. Drain the water from the pressure cooker and sprinkle the bok choy with the mustard, stirring well.

8. Cook for 2 minutes on the manual mode, then transfer the dish to the serving plate immediately.

Nutrition: calories 83, fat 4.8, fiber 2.1, carbs 7.4, protein 4.2

Sponge Bread

Prep time: 15 minutes

Cooking time: 7 minutes

Servings: 4

Ingredients:

- 1 egg

- ¾ teaspoon cream of tartar

- 1 tablespoon cream cheese

- ¾ teaspoon onion powder

- ¾ teaspoon dried cilantro

Directions:

1. Separate the egg white and egg yolk and place them into the separated bowls. Whisk the egg white with the cream of tartar until the strong peaks.

2. After this, whisk the cream cheese with the egg white until fluffy.

3. Add onion powder and dried cilantro. Stir gently.

4. After this, carefully add egg white and stir it. Scoop the mixture into the Foodi cooker to get small "clouds" and lower the crisp lid.

5. Cook the bread for 7 minutes at 360 F or until it is light brown. Chill little before serving.

Nutrition: calories 27, fat 0.2, fiber 0, carbs 0.9, protein 1.6

Pecans Rice

Prep time: 10 minutes

Cooking time: 5 minutes

Servings: 2

Ingredients:

- 1 cup cauliflower

- 1 tablespoon turmeric

- ½ teaspoon onion powder

- ½ teaspoon garlic powder

- 1 teaspoon dried dill

- ½ teaspoon salt

- 1 teaspoon butter

- 2 pecans, chopped

- ½ cup of water

Directions:

1. Chop the cauliflower roughly and place it in the food processor.

2. Pulse it for 3-4 time or until you get cauliflower rice. After this, transfer the vegetables in the cooker.

3. Add onion powder, garlic powder, dried dill, and salt.

4. Then add chopped pecans and water. Stir the mixture gently with the help of the spoon and close the lid.

5. Cook it on High-pressure mode for 5 minutes.

6. Then use quick pressure release and open the lid. Drain the water using the colander. Transfer the cauliflower rice in the big bowl, add turmeric and butter.

7. Mix up the mixture well. Serve it warm.

Nutrition: calories 145, fat 12.3, fiber 3.6, carbs 8.1, protein 3.1

Mayo Eggs

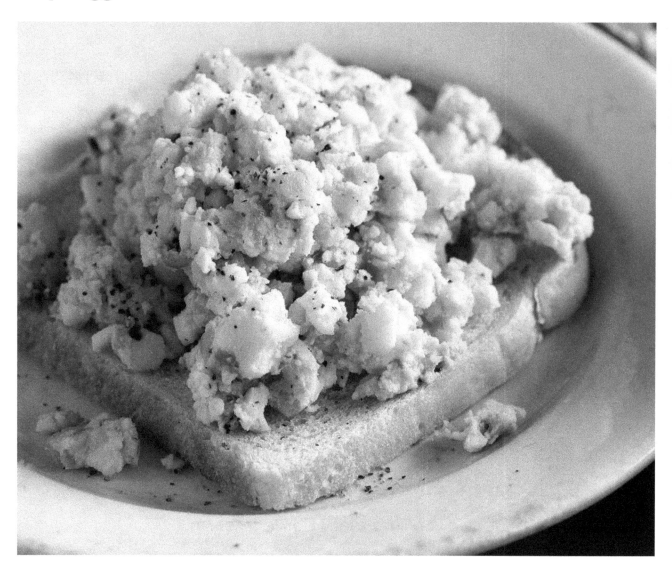

Prep time: 15 minutes

Cooking time: 5 minutes

Servings: 7

Ingredients:

- 1 tablespoon mustard

- ¼ cup cream

- 1 teaspoon salt

- 8 eggs

- 1 teaspoon mayonnaise

- ¼ cup dill

- 1 teaspoon ground white pepper

- 1 teaspoon minced garlic

Directions:

1. Put the eggs in the pressure cooker and add water. Cook the eggs at the high pressure for 5 minutes.

2. Remove the eggs from the pressure cooker and chill. Peel the eggs and cut them in half. Remove the egg yolks and mash them.

3. Add the mustard, cream, salt, mayonnaise, ground white pepper, and minced garlic to the mashed egg yolks.

21

4. Chop the dill and sprinkle the egg yolk mixture with the dill. Mix well until smooth.

5. Transfer the egg yolk mixture to a pastry bag and fill the egg whites with the yolk mixture. Serve immediately.

Nutrition: calories 170, fat 12.8, fiber 0, carbs 2.42, protein 11

Asparagus Puree

Prep time: 6 minutes

Cooking time: 6 minutes

Servings: 1

Ingredients:

- ½ cup asparagus

- ½ cup of water

- 1 tablespoon heavy cream

- 1 tablespoon fresh basil, chopped

- ½ teaspoon salt

- ¾ teaspoon lemon juice

Directions:

1. Put asparagus in the Foodi cooker. Add water and salt. Close and seal the lid.

2. Cook the vegetables on High-pressure mode for 6 minutes (use quick pressure release). Open the lid and drain half of the liquid. Add fresh basil.

3. Using the hand blender, blend the mixture until smooth.

4. Then add lemon juice and heavy cream. Stir the mash and transfer it into the serving bowls.

Nutrition: calories 67, fat 5.7, fiber 1.5, carbs 3.2, protein 1.9

Tender Salsa

Prep time: 7 minutes

Cooking time: 10 minutes

Servings: 5

Ingredients:

- 1 cup tomatoes

- 1 teaspoon cumin

- 1 teaspoon ground coriander

- 1 tablespoon cilantro

- ½ cup fresh parsley

- 1 lime

- 1 sweet green pepper

- 1 red onion

- 1 teaspoon garlic powder

- 1 teaspoon olive oil

- 5 garlic cloves

Directions:

1. Remove the seeds from the sweet green pepper and cut it in half.

2. Peel the onion and garlic cloves. Place the vegetables in the pressure cooker and sprinkle them with the ½ teaspoon of olive oil.

3. Close the lid, and set the pressure cooker to "Sauté" mode for 10 minutes. Meanwhile, chop the tomatoes and fresh parsley.

4. Peel the lime and squeeze the juice from it. Combine the lime juice with the chopped parsley, cilantro, ground coriander, and garlic powder and stir well.

5. Sprinkle the chopped tomatoes with the lime mixture.

6. Remove the vegetables from the pressure cooker.

7. Rough chop the bell pepper and onions and add the ingredients to the tomato mixture. Mix well and serve.

Nutrition: calories 38, fat 1.2, fiber 1, carbs 6.86, protein 1

Cayenne Salsa

Prep time: 10 minutes

Cooking time: 8 minutes

Servings: 6

Ingredients:

- 2 cups tomatoes

- 1 teaspoon sugar

- ⅓ cup fresh cilantro

- 2 white onions

- 1 teaspoon ground black pepper

- 1 teaspoon cayenne pepper

- ½ jalapeno pepper

- 1 teaspoon olive oil

- 1 tablespoon minced garlic

- ⅓ cup of green olives

- 1 teaspoon paprika

- ⅓ cup basil

- 1 tablespoon Erythritol

Directions:

1. Peel the onions and remove the seeds from the jalapeno pepper.

2. Transfer the vegetables to the pressure cooker and sprinkle them with the olive oil. Close the lid and cook the ingredients on the "Steam" mode for 8 minutes.

3. Meanwhile, wash the tomatoes and chop them. Place the chopped tomatoes in the bowl. Chop the cilantro.

4. Add the chopped cilantro, ground black pepper, chili pepper, and minced garlic in the chopped tomatoes.

5. Add green olives, chop them or leave them whole as desired.

6. Chop the basil and add it to the salsa mixture. Add paprika and olive oil.

7. When the vegetables are cooked, remove them from the pressure cooker and chill.

8. Chop the vegetables and add them to the salsa mixture. Sprinkle the dish with Erythritol. Mix well and serve.

Nutrition: calories 41, fat 1.1, fiber 1.9, carbs 7.7, protein 1.2

Citric Garlic

Prep time: 10 minutes

Cooking time: 9 minutes

Servings: 12

Ingredients:

- 2 cups garlic
- 1 tablespoon salt
- 1 tablespoon olive oil
- 1 teaspoon fennel seeds
- ½ teaspoon black peas
- 3 cups of water
- 5 tablespoon apple cider vinegar
- 1 teaspoon lemon juice
- 1 teaspoon lemon zest
- 1 tablespoon stevia
- 1 teaspoon red chili flakes

Directions:

1. Place the salt, olive oil. Fennel seeds, black peas, lemon juice, lemon zest, stevia, and chili flakes in the pressure cooker. Add water and stir it.

2. Preheat the liquid on the "Pressure" mode for 5 minutes. Meanwhile, peel the garlic.

3. Put the garlic into the preheated liquid.

4. Add apple cider vinegar and stir the mixture.

5. Close the lid and cook the garlic on the "Pressure" mode for 4 minutes.

6. Open the pressure cooker lid and leave the garlic in the liquid for 7 minutes, Transfer the garlic to the liquid into a glass jar, such as a Mason jar.

7. Seal the jar tightly and keep it in your refrigerator for at least 1 day before serving.

Nutrition: calories 46, fat 1.3, fiber 0.6, carbs 7.7, protein 1.5

Spicy Olives

Prep time: 10 minutes

Cooking time: 17 minutes

Servings: 7

Ingredients:

- 3 cups olives

- 1 tablespoon red chili flakes

- 1 teaspoon cilantro

- ⅓ cup olive oil

- 4 tablespoons apple cider vinegar

- 3 tablespoons minced garlic

- ⅓ cup of water

- 3 garlic cloves1-ounce bay leaf

- ¼ cup of water

- 1 teaspoon clove

- 4 tablespoons lime juice

Directions:

1. Combine the chili flakes, cilantro, apple cider vinegar, minced garlic, bay leaf, water, and lime juice together in a mixing bowl and stir the mixture.

2. Peel the garlic cloves and chop them roughly. Add the chopped garlic to the chili flake mixture and sprinkle it with the garlic.

3. Add water and place the mixture in the pressure cooker. Close the lid and cook it on the "Pressure" mode for 10 minutes.

4. Add olive oil and olives.

5. Stir the mixture well and cook it for 7 minutes.

6. When the cooking time ends, remove the mixture from the pressure cooker and transfer it to a sealed container.

7. Chill it for at least 2 hours before serving.

Nutrition: calories 186, fat 16.9, fiber 4, carbs 10.57, protein 1

Cottage Dumplings

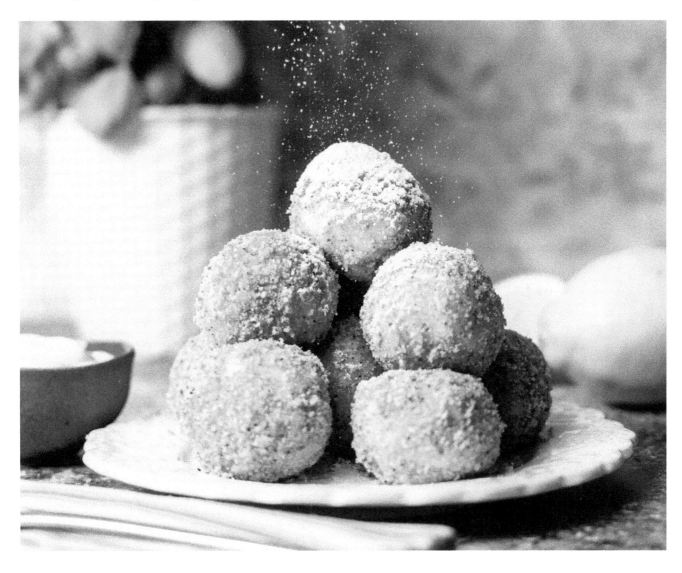

Prep time: 10 minutes

Cooking time: 15 minutes

Servings: 6

Ingredients:

- 1 cup cottage cheese

- ½ cup almond flour

- 1 teaspoon baking soda

- 1 teaspoon salt

- 2 tablespoons Erythritol

- 4 tablespoons coconut milk

- 1 teaspoon basil

- 3 eggs

Directions:

1. Blend the cottage cheese in a blender. Add eggs and continue to blend until smooth. Transfer the mixture to the bowl and add baking soda and almond flour.

2. Sprinkle the mixture with the salt, Erythritol, coconut milk, and basil. Knead the dough. Make the small logs from the dough.

3. Set the pressure cooker mode to "Steam," transfer the dough logs to the pressure cooker, and close the lid.

4. Cook for 15 minutes.

5. When the cooking time ends, remove the dumplings from the pressure cooker and serve immediately.

Nutrition: calories 102, fat 6.5, fiber 0.5, carbs 2.6, protein 8.7

Parsley Fries

Prep time: 10 minutes

Cooking time: 18 minutes

Servings: 2

Ingredients:

- 2 carrots, peeled
- 1 teaspoon salt
- 1 tablespoon olive oil
- 1 teaspoon dried parsley

Directions:

1. Cut the carrots into the fries and sprinkle with the salt and dried parsley. Mix up well and transfer them into the Foodi cooker.

2. Close the lid and cook the fries on the air crisp mode for 18 minutes (385F).

3. When the time is over, open the lid and give a good shake to fries.

4. Cook the carrot fries for a few minutes more if you want to get a crunchy crust.

Nutrition: calories 85, fat 7, fiber 1.5, carbs 6, protein 0.5

Mint Green Peas

Prep time: 10 minutes

Cooking time: 17 minutes

Servings: 5

Ingredients:

- 2 cups green peas

- ½ cup fresh mint

- 1 tablespoon dried mint

- 1 cup of water

- 1 teaspoon salt

- 1 tablespoon butter

- ½ teaspoon peppercorn

- 1 teaspoon olive oil

Directions:

1. Wash the mint and chop it. Transfer the chopped mint in the pressure cooker.

2. Add water and close the pressure cooker lid. Cook the mixture on the "Pressure" mode for 7 minutes.

3. Strain the mint leaves from the water and discard them. Add green peas, dried mint, salt, peppercorn to the liquid in the pot, and close the lid.

4. Cook the dish on the "Pressure" mode for 10 minutes. Rinse the cooked green peas in a colander.

5. Put the peas in the serving bowl and add butter and olive oil. Stir the cooked dish gently until the butter is dissolved.

Nutrition: calories 97, fat 4.6, fiber 4, carbs 11.48, protein 3

Veggie Salad with Feta

Prep time: 10 minutes

Cooking time: 15 minutes

Servings: 7

Ingredients:

- 2 medium carrots
- 7 ounces turnips
- 1 tablespoon olive oil
- 1 red onion
- 4 garlic cloves
- 5 ounces feta cheese
- 1 teaspoon butter
- 1 teaspoon onion powder
- 1 tablespoon salt
- 1 teaspoon ground black pepper
- 1 red sweet bell pepper

Directions:

1. Wash the carrots and peel them.

2. Peel the turnip, onion., and garlic cloves.

3. Put all the vegetables in the pressure cooker and cook them on the "Steam" mode for 15 minutes or until the vegetables are tender.

4. Chop the vegetables into small pieces. Combine them in a mixing bowl. Add butter and stir.

5. Sprinkle the mixture with the onion powder, salt, ground black pepper. Remove the seeds from the bell pepper and chop it.

6. Crumble the feta cheese and add all of the components to the salad. Mix carefully and serve the salad warm.

Nutrition: calories 107, fat 6.9, fiber 1.6, carbs 8.2, protein 3.8

Creamy Parmesan Casserole

Prep time: 10 minutes

Cooking time: 20 minutes

Servings: 8

Ingredients:

- 3 eggplants, chopped

- 1 white onion, chopped

- 1 bell pepper, chopped

- 1 turnip, chopped

- 1 teaspoon salt

- 1 teaspoon ground black pepper

- 1 teaspoon cayenne pepper

- ½ teaspoon white pepper

- 1 cup cream

- 5 oz Parmesan, grated

Directions:

1. Mix up together white onion, bell pepper, and turnip.

2. Add salt, ground black pepper, cayenne pepper, and white pepper. In the cooker place eggplants.

3. Then add the layers of onion mixture. Add cheese and cream.

4. Close and seal the lid.

5. Cook the casserole for 10 minutes on High-pressure mode. Then make quick pressure release. Chill the meal till the room temperature.

Nutrition: calories 144, fat 6, fiber 8.1, carbs 17.3, protein 8.5

Turnip Fries

Prep time: 15 minutes

Cooking time: 14 minutes

Servings: 5

Ingredients:

- 1-pound turnips, peeled

- 1 tablespoon avocado oil

- 1 teaspoon dried oregano

- 1 teaspoon onion powder

- ½ teaspoon salt

- 1 teaspoon turmeric

Directions:

1. Cut the turnips into the fries and sprinkle them with the dried oregano, avocado oil, onion powder, and turmeric.

2. Mix up the turnip and let it soak the spices for 5-10 minutes.

3. After this, place them in the cooker basket and close the lid. Set Air crisp mode (390F) and cook the fries for 14 minutes.

4. Stir the turnips fries twice during the cooking.

5. When the meal gets a light brown color, it is cooked. Transfer it on the serving plates and sprinkle with salt.

Nutrition: calories 34, fat 0.4, fiber 1.9, carbs 7, protein 0.9

Salty Radish

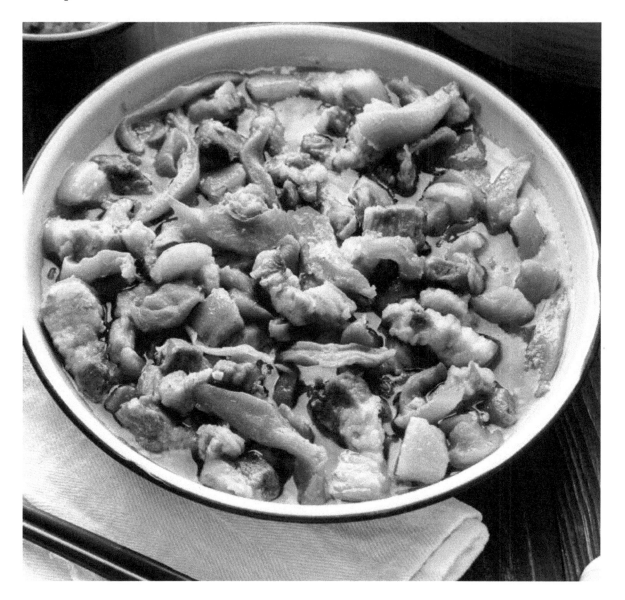

Prep time: 10 minutes

Cooking time: 8 minutes

Servings: 5

Ingredients:

- 3 cups radish, trimmed

- 1 tablespoon olive oil

- 1 tablespoon butter

- 1 teaspoon salt

- 1 teaspoon dried dill

Directions:

1. Cut the radishes into halves and place into the mixing bowl.

2. Sprinkle them with the olive oil, salt, and dried dill. Give a good shake to the vegetables.

3. After this, transfer them in the Foodi cooker and add butter.

4. Close the lid and set air crisp mode. Cook the radishes for 8 minutes at 375F. Stir the radish on half way of cooking.

5. Transfer the radishes on the serving plates and serve them hot.

Nutrition: calories 56, fat 5.2, fiber 1.1, carbs 2.5, protein 0.5

Butternut Strips

Prep time: 10 minutes

Cooking time: 15 minutes

Servings: 5

Ingredients:

- 1 pound butternut squash

- 1 teaspoon salt

- ¼ cup of water

- 2 tablespoons turmeric

- 3 tablespoons peanut oil

Directions:

1. Wash the butternut squash and peel it. Cut the butternut squash into strips.

2. Sprinkle the cubes with the salt, turmeric, and peanut oil. Stir the mixture well. Place the butternut squash strips into the pressure cooker and set it to "Sauté" mode.

3. Sauté the vegetables for 10 minutes. Stir the mixture frequently. Add water and close the pressure cooker lid.

4. Cook the dish on "Pressure" mode for 5 minutes.

5. When the cooking time ends, the butternut squash cubes should be tender but not mushy.

6. Transfer the dish to the serving plate and rest briefly before serving.

Nutrition: calories 124, fat 8.3, fiber 3, carbs 13.13, protein 1

Black Bean Pasta Salad

Prep time: 10 minutes

Cooking time: 8 minutes

Servings: 10

Ingredients:

- 8 ounces black bean pasta

- 3 cups of water

- 1 cup pork rind

- ½ cup cream cheese

- 3 medium cucumbers

- 1 teaspoon oregano

- ½ cup spinach

- 2 tomatoes

- 1 red onion

- 1 teaspoon paprika

Directions:

1. Put the pasta in the pressure cooker and add water. Close the lid and cook the pasta on "Pressure" mode for 8 minutes.

2. Rinse the pasta with hot water. Place the cooked pasta in the mixing bowl.

3. Peel the red onion and slice it. Wash the spinach and chop it.

4. Chop the tomatoes and cucumbers. Add the sliced onion, chopped spinach, tomatoes, and cucumbers in the pasta bowl.

5. Sprinkle the salad with the oregano and paprika. Add cream cheese. Blend the mixture until smooth. Add pork rind and stir the salad well.

Nutrition: calories 201, fat 9.1, fiber 6, carbs 12.7, protein 19.2

Eggplant and Onion Cubes

Prep time: 15 minutes

Cooking time: 15 minutes

Servings: 6

Ingredients:

- 3 eggplants, trimmed

- 1 tablespoon salt

- 1 tablespoon butter

- 1 teaspoon minced garlic

- 1 teaspoon onion powder

- 1 teaspoon chili flakes

- 1/3 cup heavy cream

Directions:

1. Chop the eggplants roughly and place them in the mixing bowl.

2. Sprinkle the vegetables with the salt and stir well. Leave them for 10 minutes. After this time, vegetables will give juice – drain it.

3. Transfer the eggplants in the Pressure cooker. Add butter, minced garlic, onion powder, chili flakes, and heavy cream. Mix up the mixture.

4. Cook the vegetables on Saute mode for 15 minutes.

5. Stir them from time to time. When the eggplants are tender, they are cooked.

Nutrition: calories 111, fat 4.9, fiber 9.7, carbs 16.8, protein 2.9

Cremini Puree

Prep time: 10 minutes

Cooking time: 20 minutes

Servings: 8

Ingredients:

- 12 ounces cremini mushrooms
- 3 tablespoons butter
- 1 teaspoon olive oil
- 1 big white onion
- ¼ cup cream
- 1 teaspoon salt
- 1 teaspoon ground black pepper
- 1 teaspoon chicken stock

Directions:

1. Wash the mushrooms and chop them.

2. Add the butter in the pressure cooker and melt it on "Pressure" mode. Add the chopped mushrooms and sprinkle them with salt, ground black pepper, and chicken stock.

3. Peel the onion and dice it.

4. Add the diced onion to the mushroom mixture. Sprinkle it with the olive oil and stir well.

5. Close the lid and cook the dish at "Sauté" mode for 20 minutes.

6. When the cooking time ends, transfer the mushrooms in the mixing bowl. Puree the mixture using an immersion blender.

7. Transfer the mushroom puree in the serving bowl, add cream, and mix well.

Nutrition: calories 192, fat 6.8, fiber 5, carbs 34.17, protein 5

Sweet Savory Onions

Prep time: 7 minutes

Cooking time: 15 minutes

Servings: 6

Ingredients:

- ⅓ cup liquid stevia

- 1 teaspoon of sea salt

- 1 pound white onion

- 4 tablespoons butter, unsalted

- 1 teaspoon ground ginger

- ½ teaspoon cinnamon

Directions:

1. Combine the liquid stevia and sea salt together.

2. Add ground ginger and cinnamon and stir. Peel the onion and slice it. Combine the sliced onion and stevia mixture together and mix it.

3. Leave the onions for 5 minutes.

4. Add the butter in the pressure cooker. Press the "Sauté" button on the pressure cooker. Add the onion mixture and stir gently.

5. Close the lid and cook the onions for 15 minutes. When the cooking time ends, open the pressure cooker lid, remove the onions and serve hot.

Nutrition: calories 100, fat 7.8, fiber 1.8, carbs 7.4, protein 1

Nutmeg Pumpkin Cubes

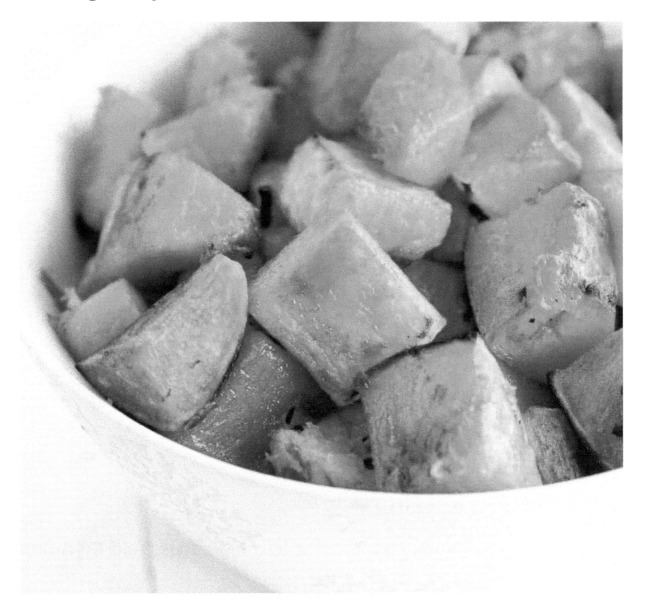

Prep time: 10 minutes

Cooking time: 10 minutes

Servings: 5

Ingredients:

- 1 pound pumpkin

- 3 tablespoons Erythritol

- 1 teaspoon ground ginger

- ¼ teaspoon nutmeg

- ½ teaspoon ground coriander

- ½ cup of water

- ½ cup sour cream

Directions:

1. Peel the pumpkin and cut it into big cubes. Add Erythritol and ginger and mix well.

2. Add nutmeg and ground coriander. Set the pumpkin aside until it releases some juice (approximately 5 minutes), then drain.

3. Transfer the pumpkin cubes in the pressure cooker and add water. Close the lid and cook the dish on the "Pressure" mode for 10 minutes.

4. When the cooking time ends, release the pressure and open the pressure cooker lid. Transfer the cooked pumpkin cubes in the serving plate and sprinkle with the sour cream.

Nutrition: calories 82, fat 5.1, fiber 2.7, carbs 8.6, protein 1.8

White Chili Onions

Prep time: 15 minutes

Cooking time: 4 minutes

Servings: 3

Ingredients:

- 2 white onions, sliced
- 1 tablespoon chili pepper
- 1 tablespoon apple cider vinegar
- 1 tablespoon olive oil
- ½ teaspoon salt
- 1 teaspoon butter
- ¾ cup of water

Directions:

1. Slice the onions and put them in the mixing bowl.

2. Add chili pepper, apple cider vinegar, olive oil, and salt. Mix up the onions well and leave them for 10 minutes to marinate.

3. After this, pour water in the cooker. Add onions and butter. Close and seal the lid. Cook the vegetables for 4 minutes on High-pressure mode.

4. Then make quick pressure release and open the lid. Stir the onions well with the help of the spoon and transfer in the serving plates.

5. The cooked vegetables should be tender but not look like a mash.

Nutrition: calories 84, fat 6.1, fiber 1.8, carbs 7.4, protein 0.9

Peppery Bok Choy

Prep time: 10 minutes

Cooking time: 8 minutes

Servings: 2

Ingredients:

- 9 oz bok choy

- 1 tablespoon olive oil

- 1 teaspoon lemon juice

- 1 teaspoon ground black pepper

Directions:

1. Wash and trim the bok choy. Cut the vegetables into halves and sprinkle with lemon juice. Transfer them in the

cooker. Add olive oil and ground black pepper. Mix up the vegetables with the help of the wooden spatula.

2. Set air crisp mode and close the lid. Cook the vegetables for 8 minutes. Stir them after 4 minutes of cooking. The cooked bok choy should have a tender texture.

Nutrition: calories 77, fat 7.3, fiber 1.3, carbs 2.8, protein 1.9

Artichoke with Creamy Sauce

Prep time: 8 minutes

Cooking time: 8 minutes

Servings: 5

Ingredients:

- 1-pound artichoke petals

- 1 cup heavy cream

- 3 oz Cheddar cheese, shredded

- 1 teaspoon minced garlic

- 1 teaspoon garlic powder

- 1 teaspoon chili flakes

- 1 teaspoon almond flour

- 1 tablespoon butter

- ½ teaspoon salt

Directions:

1. Mix up together artichoke petals, minced garlic, garlic powder, and chili flakes. Add salt. Transfer the mixture in the cooker.

2. Add shredded cheese, almond flour, and cream. Mix it up. Close and seal the lid. Cook the side dish for 8 minutes on High-pressure mode.

3. Then use quick pressure release and open the lid.

4. Mix up the artichoke petals with sauce gently and transfer into the serving bowls.

Nutrition: calories 220, fat 17.2, fiber 5, carbs 11.1, protein 7.9

Kabocha Ginger Squash

Prep time: 10 minutes

Cooking time: 2 hours

Servings: 2

Ingredients:

- 1 ½ cup kabocha squash, chopped

- ½ teaspoon ground cinnamon

- ½ teaspoon Erythritol

- 1 tablespoon butter

- ½ teaspoon ground ginger

- ½ cup of water

Directions:

1. In the cooker, mix up together kabocha squash, ground cinnamon, ginger, and Erythritol. Add butter and water.

2. Close and seal the lid.

3. Cook the vegetable on Low-pressure mode for 2 hours.

4. When the time is over and the squash is tender, transfer it in the serving bowl, add gravy from the cooker and serve.

Nutrition: calories 84, fat 5.8, fiber 1.4, carbs 7.8, protein 1.1

Thai Zucchini Strips

Prep time: 10 minutes

Cooking time: 15 minutes

Servings: 8

Ingredients:

- 3 medium green zucchini
- 1 teaspoon ground black pepper
- ½ cup of soy sauce
- 1 tablespoon sesame seeds
- 1 teaspoon salt
- ½ tablespoon Erythritol
- 1 tablespoon butter
- 1 tablespoon heavy cream
- 1 teaspoon cilantro
- 1 egg
- 1 teaspoon cumin seeds

- ½ cup almond flour

Directions:

1. Wash the zucchini and cut it into the strips.

2. Combine the ground black pepper, sesame seeds, salt, and cilantro together in a mixing bowl. Add cumin seeds.

3. Combine Erythritol and soy sauce and blend. Add the egg to the mixing bowl and whisk. Sprinkle the zucchini strips with the whisked egg.

4. Blend the mixture well using your hands. Sprinkle the zucchini strips with the almond flour, then sprinkle the zucchini with the ground black pepper mixture.

5. Add the butter to the pressure cooker and add the cream. Add the zucchini strips. Make the layer from the zucchini strips.

6. Cook the zucchini on the "Pressure" mode for 5 minutes. Remove and add a second layer of zucchini. Repeat this until all the zucchini are cooked.

7. Put the cooked zucchini strips in the pressure cooker.

8. Add the soy sauce mixture. Close the lid and sauté the dish for 3 minutes.

9. When the cooking time ends, transfer the dish to serving plates.

Nutrition: calories 61, fat 4.2, fiber 1.3, carbs 3.7, protein 2.8

Paprika Carrots

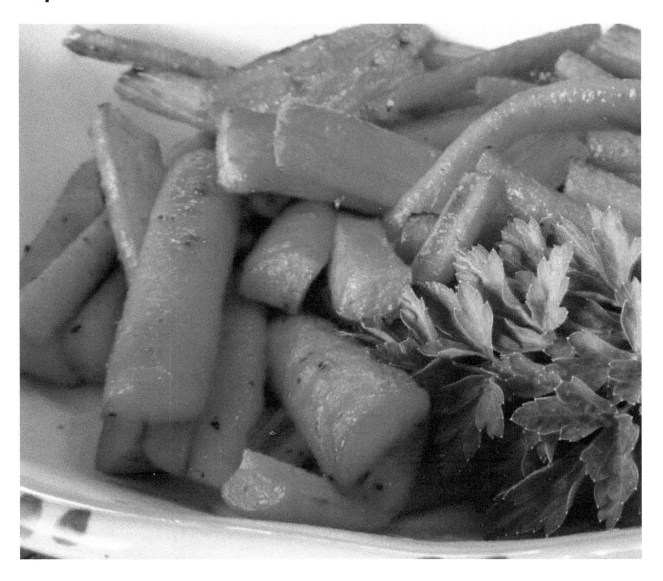

Prep time: 10 minutes

Cooking time: 10 minutes

Servings: 8

Ingredients:

- 1 pound carrots

- 9 ounces sliced bacon

- 1 teaspoon salt

- ½ teaspoon ground black pepper

- 1 teaspoon ground white pepper

- 1 teaspoon paprika

- ¼ cup chicken stock

- 1 tablespoon olive oil

- ¼ teaspoon marjoram

Directions:

1. Wash the carrot and peel it. Sprinkle the carrot with the ground black pepper.

2. Combine the salt, ground white pepper, paprika, and marjoram and stir the mixture. Coat the sliced bacon with the spice mixture.

3. Wrap the carrots in the sliced bacon. Pour the olive oil in the pressure cooker and add wrapped carrots.

4. Close the lid, set the pressure cooker to "Sauté" mode, and sauté the carrot for 10 minutes.

5. Add the chicken stock and cook the dish on the pressure mode for 8 minutes.

6. When the cooking time ends, release the pressure and open the lid. Serve warm.

Nutrition: calories 141, fat 11.4, fiber 3, carbs 7.91, protein 4

Healthy Turnip-Broccoli Mash

Prep time: 15 minutes

Cooking time: 25 minutes

Servings: 6

Ingredients:

- 8 ounces turnip

- 5 ounces broccoli

- 2 cups chicken stock

- ¼ cup cream

- 1 tablespoon salt

- 1 teaspoon cilantro

- 2 tablespoons butter

- ⅓ teaspoon thyme

Directions:

1. Peel the turnip and cut the broccoli into florets.

2. Chop the turnip and broccoli florets and place them in the pressure cooker. Add salt, cilantro, and butter and blend well.

3. Add chicken stock and close the lid. Set the pressure cooker to "Steam" mode and cook for 25 minutes.

4. When the cooking time ends, remove the vegetables from the pressure cooker. Leave a ½ cup of the liquid from the cooked vegetables.

5. Place the vegetables in a blender. Add the vegetable liquid and cream. Puree the mixture until smooth.

6. Add the butter and blend it for 2 minutes. Serve the potato-broccoli mash warm.

Nutrition: calories 62, fat 4.7, fiber 1.3, carbs 4.6, protein 1.4

Sautéed Pineapple

Prep time: 5 minutes

Cooking time: 10 minutes

Servings: 5

Ingredients:

- 9 ounces pineapple

- 1 tablespoon Erythritol

- ¼ cup lemon juice

- 3 tablespoons water

- 1 teaspoon cinnamon

- 1 teaspoon peanut oil

- ½ teaspoon paprika

Directions:

1. Peel the pineapple and cut it into the cubes.

2. Put the peanut oil in the pressure cooker. Add pineapple cubes, set the pressure cooker to "Sauté" mode, and sauté the fruit for 3 minutes, stirring frequently.

3. Add Erythritol, lemon juice, water, cinnamon, and paprika.

4. Blend the mixture gently. Close the lid and sauté the pineapple mixture for 7 minutes.

5. When the cooking time ends, remove the pineapple with the liquid from the pressure cooker. Serve it warm or chilled.

Nutrition: calories 38, fat 1.1, fiber 1.1, carbs 7.5, protein 0.4

Enoki Mix

Prep time: 10 minutes

Cooking time: 9 minutes

Servings: 4

Ingredients:

- 1-pound Enoki mushrooms

- 1 teaspoon salt

- 1 teaspoon sesame seeds

- 1 tablespoon canola oil

- 1 tablespoon apple cider vinegar

- 1 teaspoon paprika

- 1 tablespoon butter

- ½ teaspoon lemon zest

- 1 cup water for cooking

Directions:

1. Slice the mushrooms roughly and place in the cooker. Add water and salt.

2. Close and seal the lid. Cook the vegetables on High-pressure mode for 9 minutes.

3. Then allow natural pressure release. Open the lid and drain the water.

4. Transfer the mushrooms in the bowl.

5. Sprinkle them with the sesame seeds, canola oil, apple cider vinegar, paprika, butter, and lemon zest. Mix up well.

Nutrition: calories 113, fat 7.2, fiber 3.4, carbs 9.3, protein 3.2

Bell Cabbage Wedges

Prep time: 10 minutes

Cooking time: 25 minutes

Servings: 8

Ingredients:

- 10 ounces cabbage

- 3 tablespoons tomato paste

- 1 cup chicken stock

- 1 teaspoon butter

- 1 sweet bell pepper

- ¼ cup sour cream

- 1 teaspoon cilantro

- 1 teaspoon basil

- 1 medium yellow onion

Directions:

1. Wash the cabbage and cut it into the wedges. Place the cabbage wedges into the pressure cooker.

2. Combine the chicken stock, butter, tomato paste, sour cream, cilantro, and basil together in a mixing bowl and blend until smooth.

3. Peel the onion and remove seeds from the bell pepper. Chop the vegetables.

4. Add the chopped vegetables in the cabbage wedges mixture. Add chicken stock sauce and mix well using a wooden spoon or spatula.

5. Close the pressure cooker lid and cook the dish on "Pressure" mode for 25 minutes.

6. When the cooking time ends, open the pressure cooker lid and let the mixture rest briefly. Do not stir it. Transfer the dish to serving plates.

Nutrition: calories 45, fat 2.2, fiber 1.6, carbs 6, protein 1.3

Pepper Celery Stalk

Prep time: 10 minutes

Cooking time: 3 minutes

Servings: 4

Ingredients:

- 1-pound celery stalk

- 1 oz pork rind

- 1 teaspoon ground black pepper

- 1 teaspoon olive oil

- 1 teaspoon salt

- 1 cup water, for cooking

Directions:

1. Chop the celery stalk roughly and place it in the pressure cooker.

2. Add water, close and seal the lid. Cook it on High-pressure mode for 3 minutes. Then allow natural pressure release and open the lid.

3. Drain water and transfer celery stalk in the bowl.

4. Add ground black pepper, olive oil, salt, and pork rind. Mix up the ingredients well and transfer in the serving bowl (plates).

Nutrition: calories 70, fat 3.94, fiber 2, carbs 3.7, protein 5.4

Provolone Mac&Cheese

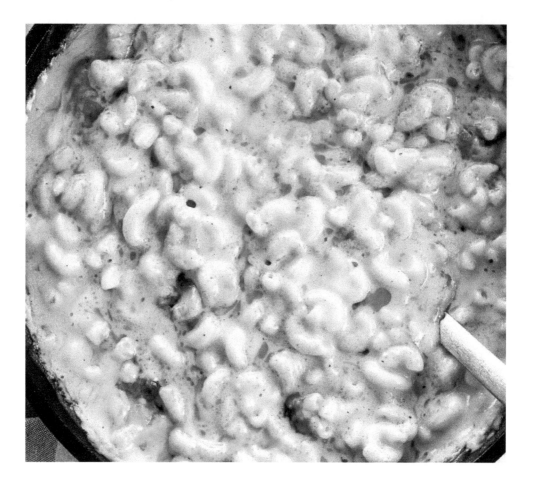

Prep time: 15 minutes

Cooking time: 5 minutes

Servings: 4

Ingredients:

- 2 cups cauliflower, shredded

- ½ cup Provolone cheese, grated

- 1 tablespoon cream cheese

- ¼ cup of coconut milk

- ¼ teaspoon salt

- ½ teaspoon white pepper

Directions:

1. Put shredded cauliflower in the instant pot bowl.

2. Top it with Provolone cheese.

3. After this, in the mixing bowl combine together cream cheese, coconut milk, salt, and white pepper.

4. Pour the liquid over the cheese and close the lid.

5. Cook the side dish on manual mode (high pressure) for 5 minutes.

6. When the time is over, allow the natural pressure release for 5 minutes more.

7. Broil the surface of the cooked meal with the help of the kitchen torch.

Nutrition value/serving: calories 114, fat 8.9, fiber 1.7, carbs 4.1, protein 5.8

Mushrooms Casserole

Prep time: 10 minutes

Cooking time: 4 hours

Ingredients:

- 1 cup Brussels sprouts, halved

- ½ cup heavy cream

- ½ teaspoon ground black pepper

- ½ cup mushrooms, sliced

- 1 teaspoon salt

- 1 oz Monterey Jack cheese, shredded

Directions:

1. In the mixing bowl combine together cheese with heavy cream, salt, and ground black pepper.

2. Place the Brussel sprouts in the instant pot in one layer.

3. Then top it with sliced mushrooms.

4. Pour the heavy cream mixture over the mushrooms and close the lid.

5. Cook the casserole on manual mode (low pressure) for 4 hours.

Nutrition value/serving: calories 120, fat 10.4, fiber 1.3, carbs 3.9, protein 4.1

Butter Mushrooms

Prep time: 5 minutes

Cooking time: 7 minutes

Servings: 2

Ingredients:

- 8 oz white mushrooms, chopped

- 1 teaspoon dried rosemary

- 2 tablespoons butter

- ½ teaspoon salt

- 1 cup chicken broth

- ¼ cup of coconut milk

- ½ teaspoon dried oregano

Directions:

1. Put mushrooms and butter in the instant pot and cook them on sauté mode for 4 minutes.

2. Then add chicken broth, dried oregano, salt, and coconut milk

3.	Close the lid and cook the side dish on manual mode (high pressure) for 3 minutes.

4.	When the time is over, make a quick pressure release.

5.	Serve the mushrooms with coconut-butter gravy.

Nutrition value/serving: calories 182, fat 13, fiber 3.4, carbs 9.8, protein 10.2

Bacon and Leek

Prep time: 10 minutes

Cooking time: 10 minutes

Servings: 6

Ingredients:

- 12 oz Brussels sprouts
- 3oz leek, chopped
- 2 oz bacon, chopped
- 1 teaspoon avocado oil
- ½ teaspoon salt
- 1 cup water, for cooking

Directions:

1. Pour water and insert the steamer rack in the instant pot.

2. Then trim Brussel sprouts and cut them into halves.

3. Arrange the vegetables in the steamer rack and cook on high pressure for 3 minutes. Then make a quick pressure release.

4. Remove the Brussel sprouts from the instant pot.

5. Clean the instant pot and rid of the steamer rack.

6. Put bacon in the instant pot.

7. Add avocado oil and cook the ingredients on sauté mode for 4 minutes. Stir them halfway of cooking.

8. Then add leek and cook the mixture for 2 minutes more.

9. Add the Brussel sprouts, mix up well and sauté the meal for 1 minute.

Nutrition value/serving: calories 85, fat 4.3, fiber 2.4, carbs 7.3, protein 5.7

Provolone Mash with Bacon

Prep time: 10 minutes

Cooking time: 8 minutes

Servings: 3

Ingredients:

- 1 oz bacon, chopped, cooked
- 1 cup spinach, chopped
- 1 tablespoon cream cheese
- ¼ teaspoon minced garlic
- ¼ cup Provolone cheese, grated
- ¼ cup heavy cream
- ¼ cup onion, diced
- ½ teaspoon white pepper
- 1 teaspoon cayenne pepper
- ½ teaspoon salt
- 1 cup water, for cooking

Directions:

1.   Put all ingredients in the instant pot baking pan.

2.   Pour water and insert the trivet in the instant pot.

3.   Place the baking pan with spinach mixture in the instant pot.

4.   Cook the dip on manual (high pressure) 8 minutes.

5.   When the time is over, allow the natural pressure release for 10 minutes and open the lid.

6.   Mix up the spinach mash carefully with the help of the spoon.

Nutrition value/serving: calories 145, fat 11.9, fiber 0.7, carbs 2.7, protein 7.3

Butter Cauliflower

Prep time: 10 minutes

Cooking time: 4 minutes

Servings: 1

Ingredients:

- 1 cup cauliflower, chopped

- ¼ teaspoon salt

- 1 tablespoon butter

- 1 cup water, for cooking

Directions:

1.   Pour water and insert the steamer rack in the instant pot.

2.   Place the chopped cauliflower on the rack and close the lid.

3.   Cook the vegetables for 4 minutes on Steam mode. When the time is over, make a quick pressure release.

4.   Transfer the cooked cauliflower in the bowl. Add butter and salt.

5.   With the help of the potato masher mash the vegetables until smooth.

6.   Add ¼ cup of water from the instant pot. If the mash is not soft enough – add more water.

7.   Mix up the mashed cauliflower well.

Nutrition value/serving: calories 127, fat 11.6, fiber 2.5, carbs 5.3, protein 2.1

Nutmeg Cauliflower Slices

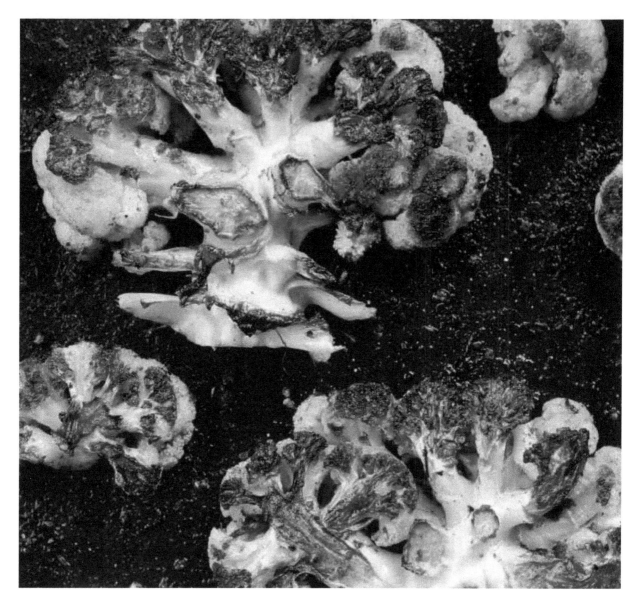

Prep time: 10 minutes

Cooking time: 5 minutes

Servings: 3

Ingredients:

- 9 oz cauliflower head, trimmed

- 1 teaspoon ground nutmeg

- ½ teaspoon ground paprika

- ½ teaspoon ground turmeric

- ½ teaspoon dried oregano

- 1 tablespoon lemon juice

- 1 tablespoon avocado oil

- ¼ teaspoon minced garlic

- 1 tablespoon heavy cream

- 1 cup water, for cooking

Directions:

1. Slice the cauliflower into the steaks.

2. Then pour water in the instant pot. Insert the steamer rack.

3. Place the cauliflower steaks on the rack and close the lid.

4. Cook the vegetables on manual mode (high pressure) for 2 minutes. Then make a quick pressure release.

5. Remove the cauliflower steaks and clean the instant pot.

6. In the shallow bowl combine together ground nutmeg, paprika, turmeric, oregano, lemon juice, avocado oil, minced garlic, and heavy cream.

7. Carefully brush the cauliflower slices with spice mixture from both side and place in the instant pot in one layer.

8. Cook the cauliflower on sauté mode for 1 minute from each side or until it light brown.

9. Repeat the same steps with remaining cauliflower slices.

Nutrition value/serving: calories 53, fat 3, fiber 2.8, carbs 6.1, protein 2

Onion Mashed Brussel Sprouts

Prep time: 10 minutes

Cooking time: 5 minutes

Servings: 4

Ingredients:

- 2 cups Brussel sprouts
- ½ teaspoon onion powder
- ¼ cup heavy cream, hot
- ¼ teaspoon salt
- 1 cup water, for cooking

Directions:

1. Pour water and insert the steamer rack in the instant pot.

2. Place the Brussel sprouts in the rack and cook it on manual mode (high pressure) for 5 minutes.

3. When the time is over, make a quick pressure release.

4.   Transfer the cooked vegetables in the food processor.

5.   Add cream, salt, and onion powder.

6.   Blend the mixture until is smooth.

7.   Put the cooked mashed Brussel sprouts in the bowls.

8.   It is recommended to serve the side dish warm or hot.

Nutrition value/serving: calories 46, fat 2.9, fiber 1.7, carbs 4.5, protein 1.7

Chicken Cauliflower Rice

Prep time: 2 minutes

Cooking time: 1 minute

Servings: 2

Ingredients:

- 1 cup cauliflower, shredded

- 5 oz chicken broth

Directions:

1. Put cauliflower and chicken broth in the instant pot.

2. Set manual mode (high pressure) and cook cauliflower for 1 minute.

3. Then make a quick pressure release. Add salt and ground black pepper if desired.

Nutrition value/serving: calories 24, fat 0.5, fiber 1.3, carbs 2.9, protein 2.4

Soft Spinach with Dill

Prep time: 5 minutes

Cooking time: 10 minutes

Servings: 2

Ingredients:

- 2 cup fresh spinach, chopped

- 1 teaspoon avocado oil

- 1 tablespoon fresh dill, chopped

- 1 teaspoon lemon juice

- ¼ teaspoon salt

- 1 teaspoon butter

- ¼ teaspoon onion powder

Directions:

1. Set instant pot on sauté mode and adjust 10 minutes.

2. Pour avocado oil and add chopped spinach.

3.   Sprinkle the greens with dill, lemon juice, salt, and onion powder.

4.   Add butter.

5.   Stir the spinach every 2 minutes.

Nutrition value/serving: calories 32, fat 2.4, fiber 1, carbs 2.4, protein 1.3

Mexican Rice

Prep time: 5 minutes

Cooking time: 4 minutes

Servings: 5

Ingredients:

- 3 cups cauliflower, shredded
- ½ teaspoon taco seasonings
- ½ teaspoon garlic powder
- 1 teaspoon lime juice
- 1 teaspoon dried cilantro
- 1 bell pepper, diced
- 2 cups chicken broth
- ½ teaspoon salt

Directions:

1. In the shallow bowl combine together taco seasonings, garlic powder, salt, and dried cilantro.

2.   Then put shredded cauliflower in the instant pot bowl.

3.   Add spice mixture.

4.   After this, add lime juice, bell pepper, and chicken broth.

5.   Gently mix up the vegetables with the help of the spoon.

6.   Close the lid of the instant pot and cook the meal on manual (high pressure) for 4 minutes.

7.   When the time is over, make a quick pressure release.

8.   Stir the side dish well.

Nutrition value/serving: calories 42, fat 0.7, fiber 1.9, carbs 6.2, protein 3.4

Pecans Parmesan Bowl

Prep time: 5 minutes

Cooking time: 10 minutes

Servings: 3

Ingredients:

- 3 pecans

- 7 oz curly kale, chopped

- 2 oz Parmesan, grated

- 2 tablespoon cream cheese

Directions:

1.   Put the pecans in the grinder and grind until you get smooth mass.

2.   Then mix up together grinded pecans with cream cheese.

3.   Heat up the instant pot on sauté mode for 2 minutes.

4.   Add cream cheese mixture and kale.

5.   Cook the ingredients for 4 minutes. Stir them halfway of cooking.

6.   Then add cheese.

7.   Cook the meal for 4 minutes more or until the kale is tender.

Nutrition value/serving: calories 214, fat 17, fiber 3.9, carbs 8.7, protein 10.9

Cabbage in Cream

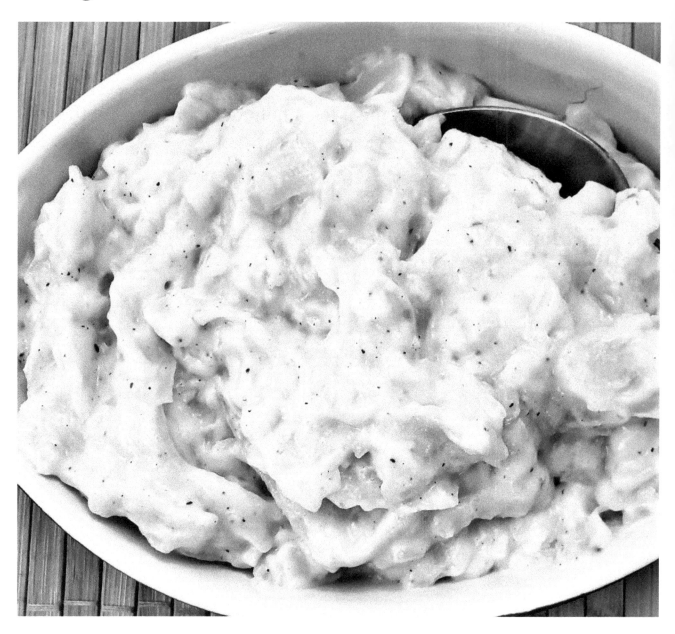

Prep time: 5 minutes

Cooking time: 7 hours

Servings: 4

Ingredients:

- 12 oz white cabbage, roughly chopped

- 1 cup cream

- 1 tablespoon cream cheese

- 1 teaspoon salt

- 1 teaspoon chili powder

Directions:

1. Put all ingredients in the instant pot bowl and close the lid.

2. Cook the vegetables for 7 minutes on manual mode (high pressure).

3. When the time is over, make a quick pressure release.

4. Open the instant pot lid and stir the cooked side dish well.

Nutrition value/serving: calories 71, fat 4.4, fiber 2.4, carbs 7.2, protein 1.8

Dill Cheese

Prep time: 5 minutes

Cooking time: 15 minutes

Servings: 2

Ingredients:

- ½ cup cauliflower, cut into florets

- ½ teaspoon dried dill

- ¼ teaspoon dried cilantro

- ¼ teaspoon dried sage

- 3 oz Parmesan, grated

- ¼ cup of organic almond milk

Directions:

1. Put cauliflower in the instant pot bowl.

2. Sprinkle it with dried dill, cilantro, and sage.

3. In the separated bowl mix up together almond milk and Parmesan.

4.   Pour the liquid over the cauliflower and close the lid.

5.   Cook the meal on sauté mode for 15 minutes. Stir the cauliflower every 5 minutes to avoid burning.

Nutrition value/serving: calories 164, fat 10.7, fiber 1.2, carbs 4, protein 14.7

Cauliflower-Tatoes

Prep time: 10 minutes

Cooking time: 5 minutes

Servings: 2

Ingredients:

- 1 teaspoon cream cheese
- ½ teaspoon salt
- ½ teaspoon ground turmeric
- ½ teaspoon white pepper
- 2 cups cauliflower
- ½ teaspoon garlic powder
- 1 cup water, for cooking

Directions:

1. Pour water and insert the trivet in the instant pot.

2. Put the cauliflower on the trivet and cook it for 5 minutes on steam mode. Then make a quick pressure release.

3.   Open the lid and transfer cooked cauliflower in the food processor.

4.   Add salt, ground turmeric, cream cheese, white pepper, and garlic powder.

5.   Then add ¾ cup of the remaining water from the instant pot.

6.   Blend the mixture until it is smooth (appx for 3-5 minutes).

Nutrition value/serving: calories 36, fat 0.8, fiber 2.8, carbs 6.6, protein 2.3

Conclusion

Being a best solution both for instantaneous pot beginners and also skilled split second pot customers this instantaneous pot recipe book raises your day-to-day food preparation. It makes you look like a professional as well as cook like a pro. Thanks to the Instant Pot part, this recipe book aids you with preparing straightforward as well as tasty meals for any kind of budget plan. Satisfy every person with passionate suppers, nutritive morning meals, sweetest desserts, and also enjoyable snacks. Despite if you cook for one or prepare bigger parts-- there's an option for any possible cooking circumstance. Improve your strategies on how to prepare in one of the most reliable method utilizing just your split second pot, this recipe book, as well as some patience to find out fast. Valuable pointers and also methods are discreetly incorporated into every recipe to make your family demand brand-new meals time and time again. Vegetarian alternatives, remedies for meat-eaters and also extremely satisfying concepts to unite the whole household at the same table. Consuming in your home is a shared experience, and also it can be so good to meet completely at the end of the day. Master your Instantaneous Pot and maximize this brand-new experience beginning today!

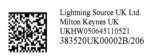

Lightning Source UK Ltd.
Milton Keynes UK
UKHW050645110521
383520UK00002B/206

9 781667 122595